When You're Ill
Or Incapacitated

Resources by James E. Miller

Books

Welcoming Change
Autumn Wisdom
The Caregiver's Book
When You Know You're Dying
One You Love Is Dying
What Will Help Me? / How Can I Help?
How Will I Get Through the Holidays?
Winter Grief, Summer Grace
A Pilgrimage Through Grief
Helping the Bereaved Celebrate the Holidays
Effective Support Groups
A Little Book for Preachers
The Rewarding Practice of Journal Writing
One You Love Has Died

Videotapes

Invincible Summer
Listen to Your Sadness
How Do I Go On?
Nothing Is Permanent Except Change
By the Waters of Babylon
We Will Remember
Gaining a Heart of Wisdom
Awaken to Hope
Be at Peace
The Natural Way of Prayer
You Shall Not Be Overcome
The Grit and Grace of Being a Caregiver
Why Yellow?
Common Bushes Afire

For additional information contact
jmiller@willowgreen.com
www.willowgreen.com

When You're Ill
Or Incapacitated

12 Things To Remember
In Times of Sickness, Injury,
Or Disability

James E. Miller

Willowgreen Publishing

This book is a collaboration in the truest sense of the word. It would not have come into being without the insight and assistance of John Aleshire, Clare Barton, Jeanna Bodart, Bob Dexter, Patricia Ferro, John Gantt, Dick Gilbert, Carrie Hackney, Gail Kittleson, Jim Kragness, Ann Lantz, Jennifer Levine, Bernie Miller, John Peterson, Micheline Sommers, and John VanderZee.

Sources cited: George Orwell, **Animal Farm**, New York, 1954; W. Somerset Maugham, **The Summing Up**, New York, 1977; and Rainer Maria Rilke, **Letters to a Young Poet**, New York, 1984.

Willowgreen Publishing
10351 Dawson's Creek Boulevard, Suite B
Fort Wayne, Indiana 46825
260-490-2222

Library of Congress Catalogue
Card Number: 95-90163

ISBN 1-885933-21-5

If you're reading this book for yourself, this is probably what you feel: you wish you felt better.

You may be grappling with an illness that has overtaken you, leaving you weakened and depleted. You may be recovering from a surgery that requires recuperation or rehabilitation. You may be trying to return to your normal self in the aftermath of an accident or another misfortune.

You may be one who has been diagnosed with a disease or a condition you will have to deal with as long as you live. Your situation may be even more serious–your life may be threatened or your future may be frightening.

<u>Where</u> you are ill or incapacitated affects <u>how</u> you are ill or incapacitated. You may be lying in a hospital bed when you read these words, or you may be in another type of healthcare facility. You may be at home or in the home of another. Every environment establishes its own limits and calls for unique responses.

You'll need to adapt the thoughts that follow for your own setting and for the changing course of your life. Some ideas will work best early in your experience, while others will be better suited for later. You'll know.

Use what will help you. Pass over what won't. Personalize this time to make it your own. Develop your own notions. Devise your own solutions.

But mostly, be receptive to what this experience can hold for you, and be open to what you can bring to this experience. Approaching it this way, you'll have little to lose, and perhaps much to gain.

1
Your feelings may be stronger than you expect, and some you may not expect at all.

Any change in your life creates stress–that's a universal law. Your stress may be minor, especially if the change is minor. Or it may feel overwhelming. Or anything in between. This unusual time may bring with it a wide variety of feelings.

A reminder: there are no "right feelings" and no "wrong feelings" for you to have. That's true for two reasons. In themselves, feelings are neither right nor wrong. They simply are. Your feelings are movements of energy flowing through you. They are an expression of your love of life, your investment in others, your natural concern for yourself.

In addition, there are no "right feelings" a person in your situation should have. Everyone is unique. No one else possesses your same history, your same personal make-up, your same experience of what's happening at the moment. What you feel, and how deeply you feel it, and how long you feel it, are individual matters.

There are certain reactions, however, that have been commonly reported during times like these. Perhaps you can identify with some of them:

• *Fear and anxiety.* You may be afraid of what you have to endure, or what your life will be like in the future, or even whether you'll have a future. You may feel at loose ends, or unusually emotional, or a bit unstable.

• *Anger.* You may feel anything from being irritable or frustrated to being downright mad. You may feel this way about your condition or about what caused your condition, about the care you're receiving or the care you're not receiving. You may be angry at family members or at friends, at medical personnel, at yourself, even at God.

• *Sadness and depression.* You may have the blues. Your days may seem grey or your future bleak. You may find yourself disturbingly low on energy.

• *Guilt.* You may feel guilty about what brought you to this point in your life. You may blame yourself for certain things that have happened, or for certain relationships, or certain attitudes.

• *Grief.* You may feel what almost everyone feels at a time like this: a sense of loss. You may grieve the loss of your health, or some physical part of yourself, or your ability to do what you've always done. You may grieve the loss of your independence, or your sense of security, or your work, or your regular relationships, or your normal routine, or your home environment. It's normal to mourn whenever you lose anything that means something to you.

Other feelings you might have include loneliness, embarrassment, or boredom. Or you may experience feelings of relief, or thanksgiving, or closeness with others, or even joy. Most likely, you will feel several of these emotions at the same time. It may be hard to sort out where one feeling ends and another begins.

Some people report feeling fragile or off balance during this time. Some even wonder if they're going a little crazy, especially when waves of unpredictable emotions wash over them time and again. Remember: this is an unusual time in your life, and unusual times call for unusual responses. That's usual.

Above all, remember that your feelings are nothing more than a sign you are human. And more importantly, they're also a sign you're nothing less than fully human. So go ahead: feel whatever it is you feel. Don't avoid your feelings, or judge them, or minimize them, or hide them. Just let them be.

2
Your feelings are designed to be expressed.

Your feelings arise from deep within. They carry valuable information about what helps you and what hinders you, what cheers you and what hurts you. Your feelings, therefore, deserve to be treated with appreciation and respect. One way to acknowledge their importance is to express them as fully as you are able.

Studies show that you tend to recuperate better and heal faster when you can release your feelings regularly. If your healing is not to be in the physical realm, expressing your feelings will still support your emotional and spiritual wholeness.

Studies also demonstrate you're likely to receive the greatest benefit by talking about your feelings with someone you value and trust. There is something therapeutic about putting what is in your heart into words so that another human being can begin to understand what you feel. You may prefer to talk with only one person in this way, or you may wish to speak with several people. It's up to you.

You may find it feels most natural to confide in one or more members of your family. You may turn to close friends. Perhaps a chaplain or social worker would be the right person if you're hospitalized, or perhaps a clergyperson or counselor would be the one if you're at home or in another setting. The best person to hear what you have to say may be someone who has undergone something similar. That's one reason why support groups are so popular.

This is not news to you: not everyone will be able to accept what you have to say. Some people are uncomfortable discussing feelings. Some do not wish to take the time. Some have not yet learned how to be good listeners. So you'll need to make sure that the person with whom you choose to share this part of yourself is a person who can be open to what you have to say.

There are other effective ways to let your feelings out. Writing them on paper or preserving them in a journal can be productive today and provide you with a helpful perspective tomorrow. You may be one who prefers to place your words on a computer screen, in which case a portable unit may be your answer.

Other ways to put words to your feelings include singing them or praying them. If you have access to a tape or CD system, you might select whatever music best captures what you feel and immerse yourself in the song or the sound.

Sometimes your feelings don't come out in words at all. They come out in groans or in tears, in sighs or in laughter. They may expend themselves as you do something physical, like hitting your pillow, or as you exert yourself in some form of exercise.

The possibilities are practically endless. You might write poetry or draw pictures, compose a painting or create a sculpture. If you're so inclined, you might play a musical instrument in such a way that when you're done playing, you've released all that's been building up inside you.

However you choose to express yourself, keep one thing in mind: it's important you be honest. Saying what you think someone else wants to hear will, in the long run, help neither of you. And forced cheerfulness at the expense of the rest of your feelings may keep others at a distance while robbing you of precious energy and needed support.

So do what will help you: express what you feel. You've been carefully designed to do just that.

3
Whatever kind of healing may be yours, more than just your physical being will be involved.

Naturally, you'd like to feel better again. You'd like to sense you are improving now or know you will improve in the future. Ideally, you'd like to be your very best.

It's possible you're healing right now from a physical illness that will one day entirely disappear. You may be recovering from a surgery that will completely solve a specific problem. You may be recuperating from an accident that will eventually leave little or no sign of what has happened to you.

It's just as possible your situation is different. You may be confronted with a condition that will never entirely disappear or with an impediment that will always shadow you. You may be learning you'll never physically recover as you wish you could. You may be realizing that your life has definite limits that it never had before.

Whatever is happening to you and whatever you are facing, you can still be on the path toward healing.

The root word for "heal" is "whole." That is its underlying meaning—"healing" is a matter of "wholing." Healing is a matter of becoming more rounded, more complete, more total. It's a process of becoming more whole as a human being.

As you already know, you are much more as a human being than just your body. Your mind, your heart, and your soul are all involved every step of the way. Sometimes that's obvious, and sometimes we tend to forget it.

Your mind plays an important role during this time, including your attitude about what has happened before and what is happening to you now. The work of your mind also includes the memories you carry, the plans you make, the ways you talk to yourself. Your heart influences this time as well, along with all your feelings and all your passions, all the bonds you have made and all the relationships you have brought to this experience. Your soul has its unique effect too, expressed in the beliefs you have formed, in the ways you practice your faith or spirituality, and in the manner you approach the deeper questions in life.

All four parts of you—your physical being, your mental being, your psychological being, and your spiritual being—have roles to play during this time of your life, just as they do in all times of your life. They complement one another. Working together, they help bring completeness to who you are as a human being.

This may sound contradictory, but it is true: whatever is happening or not happening to your body, you can still be healing. You can still be moving toward wholeness. In fact, you may be progressing toward the greatest sense of wholeness you have ever known. It's possible this experience of illness or limitation may help you see what you haven't seen before. It may give you the chance to do what you would not otherwise do.

Healing and wholeness are possible, as long as you bring all parts of yourself to this experience and as long as you are open to what the future can hold. And you can do both of those things.

4
Everyone on your medical team is of equal importance, but you are more equal than anyone.

There is this classic line in George Orwell's wonderful book, **Animal Farm**: *"All animals are equal, but some animals are more equal than others."* Obviously, despite words to the contrary, there was no equality. What was true in **Animal Farm** is also true in a certain way with your medical team. Not everyone is equal.

Your doctor has extensive training and valuable information to share with you. She or he knows things no one else on your team can know and can do things no one else can do. Your doctor may be able to save your life, literally.

Other medical personnel may serve important roles on your team: doctors who are specialists, nurses, chaplains, social workers, various therapists. One or more members of your family or circle of friends will probably be with you to represent their unique position. They can escort you to appointments, help communicate with physicians, watch over your treatment plan, boost your morale, perhaps even provide direct day-to-day care.

But never forget: you are also a central member of your own medical team. In fact, you are the central member. It's your body, your health, your future that hang in the balance. You are the only one who can truly know what is going on inside you—where your discomfort and pain are, how any medication affects you, how well any treatments are working, how your overall condition is progressing.

You do not have to be a patient patient, in the sense of compliantly waiting for people to perform their procedures on you so that you can be made well again. Your role is to actively participate in your own healing. But more than just being a full member of your team, you are the one who can exercise an authority no one else does.

You can direct your healing process in these ways:

• Express your needs, your feelings, any fears.

• Insist people use language that makes sense to you.

• Ask questions until you're sure you understand all you need to know.

• Expect to be a person who has a name, a history, and an identity apart from this illness or incapacitation. You are more than what ails you.

• Maintain your right to decide those things that are critically important to you.

• Seek second and even third medical opinions if you have serious questions.

• Rely upon your body's internal wisdom and remember it has its own timetable. Remind others, too.

• Assert your personhood with how you dress and what your room feels like, understanding there may be necessary limitations.

• Do what no one else can do for you: after you understand and once you agree, follow the directions the medical members of your team outline. Do the work required.

If there are times when it seems wise to ask another person on your team to act in your best interest, then do so. That's your right. But as much as you are able, and as often as you desire, assert your rightful authority. Build trust with every individual member of your team and with your team as a whole. Expect them to trust you, too.

Remember that you're all in this together. And remember who's in it just a little bit more.

5
Whatever is happening to you,
it's happening to people <u>other</u> than you.

No one is more affected by this episode in your life than you. No one else is touched in quite the way you are. Yet others are also affected and touched, some quite deeply.

People who love you probably understand how difficult this time can be for you. They know something of the emotions you feel, even if they cannot feel them exactly as you do. They have some idea of your struggles, even if those struggles are not exactly their own.

It's possible, of course, some of their struggles are similar to yours. If you are frightened about what the future holds for you, people who are close to you may share your same fears. If you are depressed, it may rub off on others.

Because they are as individual as you are and because their role is different from yours, your family members and friends have their own unique responses. They may feel sad or upset about what your illness or incapacitation means for them and the way they live their lives, as well as for you and the way you live yours. They may feel anxious about how well they will cope with the responsibilities that are being placed upon them. They may feel gratified they can help you.

Whether it's as simple as regular visits with you in a medical center or as far-reaching as becoming a full-time caregiver for you at home, people who assume caregiving roles with you are likely to feel stretched, if not torn. They may have other time-consuming family responsibilities to uphold. They may have jobs to maintain and employers to please. They may have worries that are unrelated to you. Or worries that are related to you.

Sometimes finances can be a bother, or much more than a bother. Sometimes treatment routines create as much havoc in their lives as in yours. Your roles may be radically changed, either temporarily or permanently. You may become more dependent than you're used to being, for instance. The other may become more decisive.

Illness and incapacitation is almost never an individual matter. It's an affair for spouses and lovers, for children and families, even for entire networks of friends and colleagues.

You can be sensitive to what others are going through by appreciating their feelings, the pressures they experience, and other obligations they must fulfill. If the timing is right and if your energy is such, you might initiate a conversation about what is happening with them. Don't second-guess what is going on with them. Ask them. Likewise, don't expect them to read your mind. Tell them.

Accept that people close to you will be making their own adjustments to what has happened to you, possibly including the realization that what has happened to you might happen to them. Don't take responsibility for them—that's counterproductive. Just try reaching out to them and let them know you are aware you're all in this together.

6
People who want to help you could use a good helper: you.

Unless you have been a caregiver yourself, you may not fully understand what people who care for you are dealing with. Some of the demands upon them have already been mentioned. They may also experience limitations.

Family members and friends who serve as your caregivers probably have had little or no training in providing convalescent care in a medical setting or at home. Their experiences with situations exactly like yours are probably rather limited, if not nonexistent. Moreover, modern healthcare trends call for more and more medical procedures to be performed in the home rather than in the hospital. As a result, inexperienced caregivers may wonder if they can handle the responsibilities your situation may require. Some tasks are not pleasant. Some medical routines are not for the squeamish.

There's another issue your helpers will face: their helplessness. However much they can do for you, there are still many things they cannot do. They cannot reverse what has happened, much as they'd like. They cannot take away any pain you might feel or other suffering you might experience. They cannot cure you.

Another difficulty your caregivers may experience–and therefore a difficulty you may experience–relates to the kind of care and the amount of care they provide. Some people don't yet understand how to be a good caregiver. There are some who may try to do too much for you, taking away your sense of personal control. They may want you to be more dependent than you're comfortable being. Others may expect you to be self-sufficient before you're quite ready.

In other words, sometimes your helpers could use some help. Here are some ideas for what you can do:

• Tell people specifically what helps you and what doesn't. That's the only way they can know for sure. Be kind, be patient, but be clear.

• Let people know when you appreciate specific things they do for you. Positive reinforcement succeeds.

• Do as much for yourself as seems appropriate. Don't overdo, but also don't give in to the temptation of expecting people to wait on you any longer than is good for all of you.

• Be aware of people's limitations. Avoid asking someone to do what they're not ready or able to do. See if someone else is available.

• Appreciate that your caregivers need to care for themselves. Help them feel good about getting their own rest. Encourage them to do things they enjoy and to spend time with others, if they wish.

• Treat this caregiving relationship as a care-sharing relationship. Offer your caregivers whatever it is you have to give them. Perhaps it's your moral support, or your sense of humor, or your understanding acceptance, or your interest in their lives, or all these things.

• Remember that one way your caregivers deal with their sense of helplessness is by doing whatever they can for you. Be understanding of that tendency. If their hovering feels excessive, talk about it, including why they might be acting that way.

You are being given the opportunity to draw close to other human beings in what can be a truly reciprocal relationship. You each have something to give and you each have something to receive. So give what you can and receive as you'd like. As you do so, you can model what good helping is all about.

7
However hard it may be for you, this is a time to take it easy.

If you're like many people, several platitudes have been engrained within you: "Keep busy." "Work hard." "Be productive." Then there come episodes in your life like this one which may call into question the usefulness of those words. It's difficult to feel productive when you're ill or incapacitated. It's hard to keep busy when you're confined to bed.

Ignoring those messages about working hard is not easy work. You have lived your life a long time under the influence of such advice. Perhaps too long. You may have tied much of your value as a person to what you have been able to accomplish. Perhaps too much.

The rules are now suspended. Here are the new ones in their place: "Relax." "Be gentle with yourself." "Take your time."

Above all else, this is a time to take things easy. Your body needs rest to do what it is meant to do. So you will do well to give it what it calls for. When you're tired, lie down. When you're sleepy, doze. When you feel quiet, be silent.

This may be a good time to learn a technique or two for calming your body and your mind. A common one is to lie comfortably and to "talk" to different parts of your body, encouraging each one to relax. While doing this, breathe slowly and deeply. Begin with your toes, your feet, your calves and move slowly all the way up your body to your head. You might read about other methods of mental imagery that can help you or speak with someone who is knowledgeable about relaxation techniques.

You may choose to make this time relaxing in other ways. You might try various kinds of soothing music, or an audiotape or videotape that leads you into quiet meditation.

Learning to be easier with yourself can help you be easy with others. You can learn to give them the same flexibility you yourself deserve. You can let strict schedules slide a little. You can lower unnecessarily high expectations.

This may be an important time for you to take it easy in an even deeper way. Perhaps you have let certain rigid ideas or routines become driving influences on your life. Common examples are the notions that we always have to "look good" or that we need to possess "perfect health." Is this a good time to re-think such notions?

Perhaps there are ways you have automatically responded to particular people in the past, or barriers you have placed between yourself and others. Perhaps from this new vantage point you can see how limiting this has been. Is this a good time to let go of those patterns?

It may be that forgiveness is an issue for you. Maybe you'll want to forgive your body for "betraying" you. Maybe you'll find meaning in forgiving others for what they have done to you. Maybe you'll discover it's you who needs the forgiveness, either for what you have done or for what you haven't done. Maybe it's all on a grander scale—maybe you're ready to forgive the world, and everything in it, for not being perfect.

Whatever is happening in your life these days, it's a good time to relax and to mellow. It's a good time to be less concerned about doing and more open to just being. It's a perfect time to take it easy.

8
You may find value in asking of this time, "What am I being told?".

Sometimes things do not happen without reason. Causes lead to effects.

Sometimes you can see patterns developing in your life that you've never noticed before.

Sometimes random happenings are suddenly seen for what they are: not random at all.

The issue here is not about finding the meaning of this time in your life. It's simpler than that. It's merely a matter of looking more closely at these events and asking, "Is something going on here I should notice?".

There are no surefire ways every person can use to search for these messages. A general rule, however, is that an open, curious mind that looks beyond the obvious often makes interesting discoveries. An inquiring soul that can step back far enough to see the larger picture can be rewarded with valuable insight.

You might pose a few questions about events leading up to this episode:

What were the direct causes?

What, or who, caused the causes?

Did my lifestyle choices contribute to what has happened? If so, which ones? If so, what is the message?

Have others been telling me something I am just now able to hear?

You might ask questions of the episode itself:

Why is this happening now rather than another time?

Why is this happening to me and not someone else?

Is there an obvious reason this particular part of my body is involved? Is there a reason that isn't so obvious?

Is there something in my life I have been unhappy about? If so, is that related to what is going on now?

What happens to my lifestyle or my work as a result of this episode, and how do I feel about that?

What is happening to my relationships with those closest to me, and how do I feel about that?

Is there something I am trying to escape?

How do I feel about the kind of attention I am getting?

Spending a little time with questions like these may yield interesting information. One man came to see that he used his illnesses as a way to get much-needed attention. A woman professional realized the only way she could give herself permission to take time off work was to have a health crisis, and she had one about every two years. Another came to see that a recurring skin condition related to more than just her skin; it related to her self-concept.

When you put answers to the question, "What am I being told?", try on each answer several times before accepting it. You might want to talk over your thoughts with someone who knows you, someone you trust.

There is one more important fact to consider when you pose this question—it's entirely possible that nothing at all is being told you. Quite often happenings are only that: happenings. It's unfair to yourself to read into them an underlying message that isn't there.

So take your time, be honest, and be thorough. Listen carefully, and if something is being said, you'll figure it out. And if nothing is being said, you'll figure that out, too.

9
This serious time is best approached
with a sense of humor.

What has happened to you is no laughing matter. If you are suffering, if your future is clouded, if you feel lonely or depressed, you are not inclined to look on the lighter side.

Let's be clear: you should not deny your emotions. If you feel low, pretending otherwise will only put you out of touch with yourself and with others. But let's be equally clear about this: it's possible to be ill and still find things to feel good about. It's possible to be going through a darker period of your life and still find moments of brightness. It's possible to know sadness and still find something to laugh about.

These are not empty words. One of the saddest times of my life was when my wife developed breast cancer and underwent surgery and chemotherapy. For a long time we felt shadowed by a great, dark cloud. Yet even in the midst of that anguish and fear, we still found things to laugh about. Sometimes we were intentional in finding the humor, and it worked—we found it. But sometimes the humor found us, even without our trying. Never have we known such joy in the midst of such sorrow.

You can know joy, too. You can choose to approach this time with the belief you can still enjoy people around you. It can show in the way you greet them and how you speak with them. It can reveal itself in the choice of your words and with the look on your face. It can surface in your readiness to be amused.

Perhaps you can find humor in the ordinary routines of your day or in the unexpected mix-ups of your life. Maybe it's yourself you can take lightly, or your hospital garb, or that medical procedure that is as embarrassing to your modesty as it is essential to your health.

You can invite people to bring their jokes to you, and

you can enliven your time with them by telling your own. You can watch TV shows or movies that tickle your funny bone. You can read articles or books that make you smile, or return again to those get well cards that bring out a chuckle. You can turn to those people who have always been able to cheer you and invite them to spend time at your side.

Laughing can divert your attention, and it can help you see things from another perspective. Research is even showing that laughter can be good for you medically. It causes the release of powerful natural pain relievers in your brain. It can increase the immune response of your body. It can help get more oxygen to your blood. In other words, it can help you physically.

Another benefit is that humorous experiences can cheer you more than once. You are lifted when you laugh and you hear the laughter of others. You are lifted again each time you remember the laughter, and each time you pass the story of it along.

You'll want to remember that people will be taking their cues from you. If they sense you're not open to lightheartedness, they'll hold back. Of course, sometimes you won't be in the mood for joking. But at other times perhaps you will be. When you are, let people know.

Claim the kind of humor that works best for you. It may be light or dark. It may come out as giggles or as guffaws. But whatever you do, don't let opportunities for happiness, however small, pass you by without at least giving them one of your winks. And if you want, you can even burst out laughing.

10
You have the resources to do
what you have been given to do.

Your illness or disablement may be a nuisance to you. It may be a problem for you to solve or a hurdle for you to overcome. On the other hand, your experience may be much more serious than that. You may be wondering how you will possibly make it through this time. You may be doubting if you have what it takes to do what it appears you must do. In your wonderings, remember these facts:

• *You have been a survivor in the past.* This is not the first difficulty you have known or the only life crisis you have endured. Like all human beings, you have struggled. But you have done more than struggle. You have persevered. You have learned. Chances are you have triumphed. What you have done in the past you can do again. Perhaps today's arena is different. Perhaps you have never taken on what is presently waiting for you. Still, you do have experiences and talents that have served you well in the past. They can yet again.

• *You possess coping skills today.* Your daily life is made up of changing situations you must address and inconveniences you must accommodate. Things do not always go as predicted or as expected. One must learn to adapt, and you have—otherwise you would not have come this far. Whatever coping skills you have, you can use them to adjust to this situation. Whatever you know about managing stress, about making transitions, about dealing with loss, and about a host of other subjects, you can use those skills today. And you can expand upon them and learn still more. Teachers are always nearby.

• *You are blessed with professional support.* Your doctors, nurses, therapists, chaplains, and other health-related professionals stand ready to offer not just their knowledge and expertise, but their sensitivity and compassion as well. People who choose this kind of work usually approach it more as a calling than as a career. They want to help and they are uniquely qualified to do just that. They can be a blessing.

• *You are surrounded by personal support.* Most likely, you have family or friends who can often be with you when you need them. Most likely, you have their unquestioned dedication and their unspoken affection (and, if you're fortunate, you'll have their spoken affection, too). But even if those nearest and dearest to you are not quite near or dear enough, you can still find others to lean on. You may find a helping hand or a listening ear in the next bed, or the next room, or next door. You may find support by joining a like-minded group of people or by opening yourself to the assistance of your congregation, a social organization, or a volunteer agency. Help is waiting.

• *You have internal resources at your disposal.* While you may know fear, you also know courage. While you may sometimes doubt, you also have faith. While you may wonder, you can also hope. One of your greatest resources can be the way you focus your thoughts. You can choose what your attitude will be—whether this experience will be viewed as a catastrophe or as a challenge, whether you will see yourself as a victim or as a free person, whether you will be only diminished by this event or somehow enriched. What you have within you is very powerful.

• *You are upheld by what you cannot see.* Others can hold you in their wishes and by their prayers. Souls can connect across all barriers of time and space. And whether it is apparent to you or not, there is an Abiding Presence in the mystery all around. You are not alone. You are upheld.

11
You can use this time for all it's worth, and it can be worth a great deal.

The writer W. Somerset Maugham was once confined to bed in a tuberculosis sanitarium. He later wrote of that time,

"For the next two years I led an invalid life. I had a grand time. I discovered for the first time in my life how very delightful it is to lie in bed. It is astonishing how varied life can be when you stay in bed all day and how much you find to do."

His words sound unreasonably cheerful. Two years quarantined in bed with a serious illness as "a grand time"? However difficult it might be to duplicate his feelings, there is something to be said for the thought he expressed: a time of illness or the experience of incapacitation can also be a period of exploration, of appreciation, and of growth.

• *This can be a time away.* In a sense this experience is a journey to another space. Calling it a vacation would be terribly inaccurate, yet it does contain some of the very characteristics a vacation holds. This is an interlude from your regular duties and responsibilities. It is a sanctioned time off when rest is encouraged. It is a break which can give you a change of scenery and the chance to "recharge your batteries."

• *This can be a time alone.* You may be a person who needs a great deal of solitary time, or you may seek it in only small doses. But you need at least some—everyone does. This experience can help fulfill that urge. There is also something to be said for making the most of your time alone even when you don't want that kind of time. There are lessons to be learned about how the discomfort of loneliness can turn into the comfort of solitude. This can be a time to develop a close and lasting friendship with someone very important: yourself.

• *This can be a time of togetherness.* People are concerned about you and will show it. Some will want to be close to you. Others may want to do things for you. The sense of concern, community, and camaraderie can be life-giving.

• *This can be a time of savoring.* What you are being given is a series of present moments. Perhaps you can learn to cultivate an appreciation for what all present moments hold: things like shapes and colors you often don't take time to see, or sounds and voices you usually don't take time to really listen to. Tastes and aromas are always waiting for you. So is the complete sensation of touch. You can connect with the world around you in a way you won't soon forget.

• *This can be a time of the eternal.* The conditions which times like this may impose are similar to the conditions religious disciplines call for: abstinence, stillness, isolation. So this time might become for you a ready-made retreat. Because of the leisure you have and because of the issues you face, you can make this a period of meaningful reflection, if you so choose. Some people report they turn naturally to prayer and meditation at these times. Others find prayer to be difficult due to pain or discomfort. If that is your experience, perhaps someone will pray with you, translating what is in your heart and soul into words. Some wish to return to favorite religious texts for hope and encouragement, while others discover an urge to delve into such readings for the first time. Some find what feeds them in music or in poetry or in quiet sharing with another.

Whatever you make of this time, there is much to be made of it. It's up to you.

12
This experience holds the potential
for you to discover your own deep meaning.

There is an old Chinese story about a farmer who was tilling his field with his only horse when it bolted and disappeared into the hills. The farmer's neighbors gathered around him, offering their sympathy for his misfortune. His response was, "Misfortune? We'll see." A week later the horse returned, bringing with it a herd of wild stallions. This time the neighbors congratulated him on his good fortune. He responded, "Good fortune? We'll see." Several weeks later the farmer's son, attempting to tame one of the wild horses, fell and broke his leg very badly. Neighbors offered their condolences and the farmer said, "We'll see." Not long after, the army marched into the village, taking with them every able-bodied young man they could find. The farmer's son, his leg in a splint, was allowed to remain in the safety of his home. Once again, the farmer's apparent misfortune turned into fortune.

As it was with the Chinese farmer, so it is with you and with me. When we ask, "What is the meaning of this unwanted incapacitation?", will we have the patience to wait, and to ponder, and to be open to what life is giving us? Will we be able to say "We'll see," and then work at really seeing?

The German poet Rainer Maria Rilke once wrote in a letter to a young man who had complained about the effects of illness on his life:

> *"Why do you want to shut out of your life*
> *any agitation, any pain, any melancholy,*
> *since you really do not know what those*
> *states are working upon you?"*

Is there any possibility this could be true in your life? Is there any way your illness or accident or disablement is somehow working upon you in a way that is positive, however hard that may be to see? Do you have any sense you are learning something important about yourself, or about others, or about life? Is there any way your inner strength is being deepened, if ever so slightly? Is your wisdom growing, if ever so slowly? What about your courage? Your compassion? Your conviction?

Is it possible you're learning valuable information about what your priorities have been so you can re-decide what you want them to be? Do you sense this experience can help you re-align your life so that you're more in touch with yourself, with others, with the world?

In other words, do you have any opportunities here, however hidden or however small? Do you see that your life can somehow become enlarged, whatever is happening to your body? Can you become more fulfilled, whatever your limits? Can you be gaining, despite what you are losing, and perhaps even because of it? Can something new in your life begin, even as something else ends?

Whatever meaning you are starting to make of this period of your life, know that this meaning is yours and yours alone. Its significance is quite personal. Its truth is quite original. And its value depends upon what you will do with it. The decision is yours.

A Final Word ...

What is happening to you right now is changing you. You will not be the same.

Your changes may be minor. You may resume your routines with a minimum of inconvenience and go about your life much as before. But your life won't be exactly like it was. Certain memories will remain. Certain warnings will linger. Certain lessons will not be forgotten.

It's possible your changes will be major. Life may assume a whole new dimension. And so may you. Something may be taken from you, while perhaps something else will be given. Something may be laid on you, while perhaps something else is lifted. You may be hurt and healed in the same moment.

This much is sure: what will be made of these changes, for the greatest part, is up to you.

Others can be with you, but they cannot step into your place.

Others can help you, but they cannot do it for you.

Only you can persevere. Only you can change. Only you can heal.

But the good news is that you <u>can</u>. You can, because you have in the past. You can, because others have done so before you and they have shown the way. You can, because others are in similar situations right now, ready to share what they know. You can, because there are people who care for you as much as you care for yourself.

No, your life will not be the same. It can be better.

An Affirmation for Those Who Hurt

The undeniable truth is this:
*   physical suffering is a condition of life on earth.*
No one is forever exempt.
There is an affliction to illness and disease
*   that narrows one's vision and diminishes one's vitality.*
There is a wounding to physical trauma of all sorts
*   that can hurt not just one's body but one's spirit as well.*
There can be a torture to life-changing disablement
*   and an agony to life-threatening disease*
*   that can darken one's days and blacken one's nights.*
Yet I believe that suffering can be more than mere suffering,
*   and pain can be a pathway leading beyond itself*
*   to something of abiding significance.*
For that which hurts and limits can be just as well
*   that which refines and instructs.*
What is refined is one's wisdom, one's courage, one's endurance.
What is instructed is one's understanding of the paradoxes of life:
*   what starts with breaking down can end with building up;*
*   what originates with loss can terminate with gain;*
*   what begins in fear can come to its conclusion with love.*
And then times of aching can be turned into times of healing,
*   as struggle gives way to awareness and acceptance,*
*   as limitation yields to a new sense of freedom and openness.*
When that happens,
*   those who suffer can become those who are renewed,*
*   and those who grieve can become those who are transformed.*
I believe this not only can *happen but it* does *happen.*
I believe it happens here as easily as anywhere.
I believe it happens now as readily as any other time.
I believe it happens with a design and with a purpose all its own,
*   and it is not apart from us, but we are a part of it.*
And we are a part of It.
*   —James E. Miller*

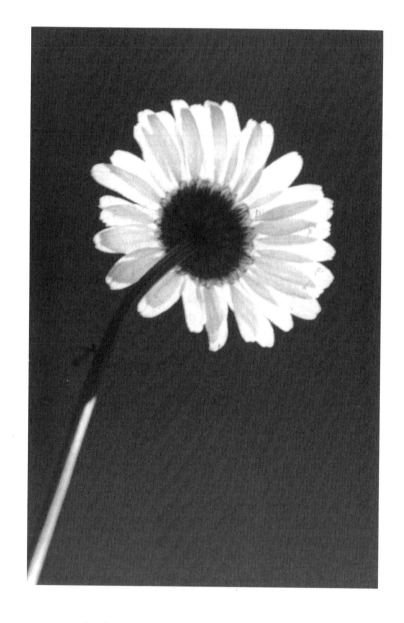

Remember that whatever is happening to you, this time of your life
can be a time of becoming more whole, if you wish it to be.